TIRED OF
BEING TEASED
OBESITY AND OTHERS

OBESITY & KIDS

TIRED OF
BEING TEASED
OBESITY AND OTHERS

BY JAMIE HUNT

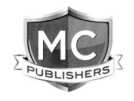

Mason Crest Publishers

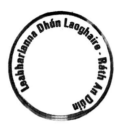

MASON CREST PUBLISHERS INC.
370 Reed Road
Broomall, Pennsylvania 19008
(866)MCP-BOOK (toll free)
www.masoncrest.com

First Printing
9 8 7 6 5 4 3 2 1

ISBN (set): 978-1-4222-1705-4
ISBN: 978-1-4222-1711-5

Library of Congress Cataloging-in-Publication Data

Hunt, Jamie.
  Tired of being teased : obesity and others / Jamie Hunt.
      p. cm. — (Obesity & kids)
  Includes bibliographical references and index.
   ISBN 978-1-4222-1711-5 (hardcover)   ISBN 978-1-4222-1705-4 (hardcover series)
   ISBN 978-1-4222-1899-0 (pbk.)   ISBN 978-1-4222-1893-8 (pbk series)

  1. Obesity in children—Juvenile literature. I. Title.
  RJ399.C6H86 2010
  618.92'398—dc22

2010012759

Design by Wendy Arakawa.
Produced by Harding House Publishing Service, Inc.
www.hardinghousepages.com
Cover design by Torque Advertising and Design.
Printed in USA by Bang Printing.

The creators of this book have made every effort to provide accurate information, but it should not be used as a substitute for the help and services of trained professionals.

CONTENTS

INTRODUCTION FOR THE TEACHERS

We as a society often reserve our harshest criticism for those conditions we understand the least. Such is the case for obesity. Obesity is a chronic and often-fatal disease that accounts for 400,000 deaths each year. It is second only to smoking as a cause of premature death in the United States. People suffering from obesity need understanding, support, and medical assistance. Yet what they often receive is scorn.

Today, children are the fastest growing segment of the obese population in the United States. This constitutes a public health crisis of enormous proportions. Living with childhood obesity affects self-esteem, which down the road can affect employment and attainment of higher education. But childhood obesity is much more than a social stigma. It has serious health consequences.

Childhood obesity increases the risk for poor health in adulthood—but also even during childhood. Depression, diabetes, asthma, gallstones, orthopedic diseases, and other obesity-related conditions are all on the rise in children. Recent estimates suggest that 30 to 50 percent of children born in 2000 will develop type 2 diabetes mellitus, a leading cause of preventable blindness, kidney failure, heart disease, stroke, and amputations. Obesity is undoubtedly the most pressing nutritional disorder among young people today.

If we are to reverse obesity's current trend, there must be family, community, and national objectives promoting healthy eating and exercise. As a nation, we must demand broad-based public-health initiatives to limit TV watching, curtail junk food advertising toward children, and promote physical activity. More than rhetoric, these need to be our rallying cry. Anything short of this will eventually fail, and within our lifetime obesity will become the leading cause of death in the United States if not in the world. This series is an excellent first step in battling the obesity crisis by educating young children about the risks, the realities, and what they can do to build healthy lifestyles right now.

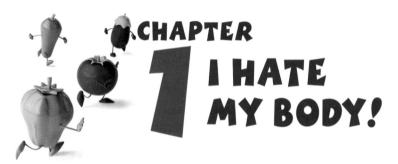

CHAPTER 1
I HATE MY BODY!

"Why can't I look like Sierra?" Patti wailed. "I hate myself."

Patti stared at her reflection in the changing room mirror. The one-piece bathing suit her mother had picked out for her clung to her bulging belly and rode up over her round bottom. "I look like a baby whale," Patti announced. Her voice quavered as she said the words, and she sniffed back the tears that were trying to get out.

"You do not," her mother said firmly. "You have a very pretty face. And you're solid."

The tears Patti had been holding back spilled over. She had heard those words so many times in her ten years of life:

Looking in the mirror can be hard if you are not happy with the person looking back at you.

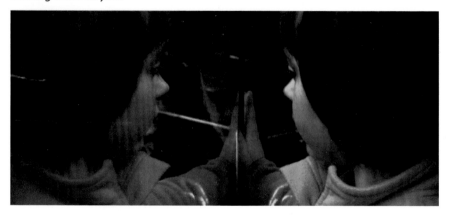

"You're so solid, Patti." "Husky," was the word her grandma used. Her aunt Terri said she was "chunky." But all those words just meant "fat." And having a pretty face was like the consolation prize they hand out to the person who comes in last, a lame complement that was supposed to make her feel better, when all it did was say one more time, "You, Patti Garcia, are fat!"

Meanwhile, her sister Sierra was as skinny as a string. She was two years older than Patti—but while Patti at ten was already wearing a LARGE in adult woman sizes, Sierra could still fit into the same shorts and bathing suits she had worn when she was seven years old. Their mom had just bought Sierra an adult size dress, but it was extra-small petite size. Sierra looked beautiful in it.

Sierra always looked beautiful. And no matter what Patti wore, she always looked like a whale.

DID YOU KNOW?

A stereotype is a picture we have in our heads about a group of people. It's not necessarily true. In fact, it seldom is, because people are individuals, and each person within a group is different. But many people have a stereotype in their heads when they think about people who are overweight and obese. Thinking of people who are overweight as "pigs" is just part of that stereotype—but pigs are also the victims of untrue stereotypes. In reality, pigs are not normally fat. If they have their choice, they are not normally dirty. And pigs are very intelligent. So remember: stereotypes are often simply not true!

Boys liked to look at Sierra. The same boys made fun of Patti and called her "Fatty Garcia."

Sierra was normal. Patti was weird.

Patti loved her sister, but sometimes she felt like she hated her too.

But she didn't really hate Sierra. She stared in the mirror at the tears rolling down her round cheeks. "I hate myself," she repeated. "I hate my body."

THE OBESITY PROBLEM

Patti Garcia feels as thought she's weird because she's overweight, but the reality is that she's not weird at all. More people today, including children, are overweight and **obese** than at any other time in history.

Countries all around the world have begun to worry about the obesity problem. In America, nearly two out of every three adults are overweight, and one out of three adults are obese. One out of every six children are overweight. In the past thirty

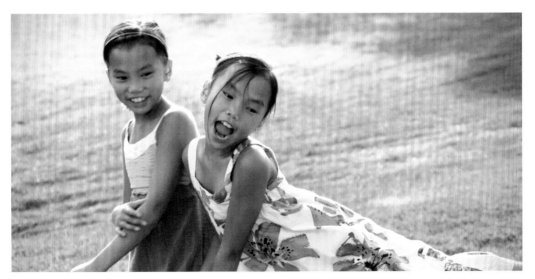

Sisters often have a very close and loving relationship, but competition and feelings of jealousy are also common.

years, the number of obese preschoolers has doubled, and around the world, there are over 42 million overweight pre-schoolers! Meanwhile, there are three times as many school-age children who are obese as there were back in 1980.

Being overweight puts these children at risk of getting sick. Being overweight or obese also makes it more likely that these children will grow up to be obese or overweight adults—which will mean that they may get other diseases when they grow up.

What does obese mean? It means to have much more body fat than is normal or healthy. It's considered to more serious than being overweight.

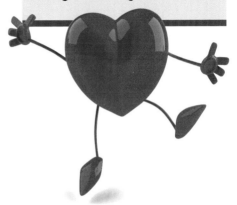

Obesity is a big health problem, and the whole world is facing it.

So Patti's not alone, and she's not weird. But Patti is facing another problem besides being overweight. Patti hates her body. And that's a big problem.

BODY HATE

Being overweight isn't healthy. But hating your body isn't healthy either.

No matter what you look like, your body is amazing. Think about it. Your brain is more complicated than a

This chart shows how common obesity is among adults in the United States. The data includes Washington, D.C

Percent of Obesity in U.S. Adults	
15% to 19%	1 State
20% to 24%	20 States
25% to 29%	27 States
More than 30%	3 States

computer—and it works faster and better than any computer. Your eyes and ears take in light and vibrations, and then send messages to your brain, allowing you to see and hear. Your heart beats over and over and over, never resting for seventy, eighty, even one hundred years, sending blood through your veins every second of every day. Every moment, your body does all the complicated jobs that not only keep you alive but that also allow you to think, feel, talk, learn, play, laugh, cry, dream, and work. If you stop to really think about it, you're realize your body is a miracle. It takes in food and turns it into energy. It breathes in oxygen and sends it out to each of the tiny cells in your body. It's more magic than any wizard's spell!

But many people in the world today feel like Patti does. They don't realize how wonderful their own bodies are. They criticize other people's bodies. They don't give their own bodies the love and respect they deserve. Instead, they hate their bodies—or they're not kind to others whose bodies are overweight or obese. They make judgments about how nice or smart or interesting other people

are based on what they look like. And they turn this same mean attitude against themselves.

Many things teach us we should look a certain way. Magazines, television shows, movies, and commercials all show us gorgeous models and actors who never have an ounce of fat on their bodies. Even little children

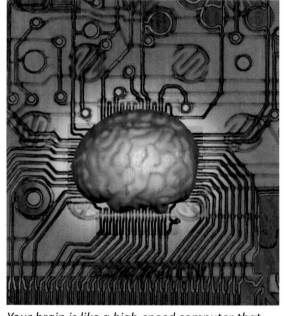

Your brain is like a high-speed computer that controls the rest of your incredible body.

quickly pick up the message that if they want to be pretty or good-looking, they need to look the same way: skinny! The companies that make diet pills and other products to help you lose weight send out constant messages through advertisements and commercials: You need to lose weight! (So buy our product.)

Prejudice is the word we use when we think differently about others because of their race, their religion, or the way we look. Most of us know that this is wrong—but many people think it's okay to think about people differently because they are overweight or obese. This is a form of prejudice too. And yet we hear fat jokes at school all the time. Grownups tell fat jokes too. People on television do as well. Most of the time, people forget how cruel this is, or how it makes others feel.

So as many of us get fatter and fatter, we also become more and more convinced that the only way for us to be beautiful, to be respected, to be admired by others is to be thin. It's a situation that makes many people miserable.

What are researchers? They're people who study and do tests to find out the answers to questions.

Researchers have found that eight out of every ten children are worried about being fat. Nearly half of all first- and third-graders said they wanted to be thinner. These children may grow up to hate their bodies.

People who hate themselves and their bodies don't take as good care of themselves. They're more likely to be **depressed**. They may withdraw from others. They may not have the confidence in themselves they need to do well in life. As a result, they may have problems in school or in the work world. It may be harder for them to make friends and get along with others.

What does it mean to be depressed? Someone who is depressed is sad most of the time. Everyone feels sad sometimes, a person who is depressed feels sad every day.

And guess what? All those problems may also mean they turn to food to help them feel better. So it's like a circle, where one problem just feeds into the other, and they both get worse and worse.

When that happens, we need to find a way to break the circle.

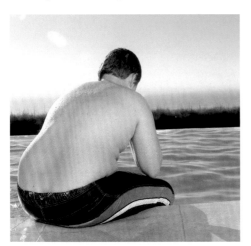

Children who are overweight may get teased until they no longer like to be around other people.

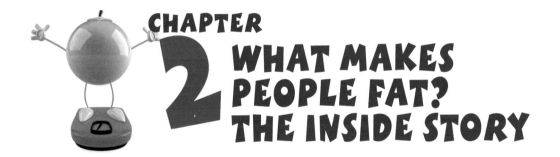

CHAPTER 2
WHAT MAKES PEOPLE FAT? THE INSIDE STORY

"You're a fat lazy slob!" Sierra screamed at her sister. "Why can't you keep your side of the room picked up? I'm tired of tripping over your dirty clothes."

Patti stared at her sister. She and Sierra usually got along. The only thing they fought over was the bedroom they shared. Patti's side of the room was by the door, Sierra's was by the window, so Sierra had to walk through Patti's side to get to hers. And Patti's side was always a mess. She knew it bugged Sierra, but most of the time, she didn't really care. She liked her side of the room the way it was. She had better things to do than hang up her clothes.

But Sierra had never before told her she was fat. Patti burst into tears. She picked up her pillow and heaved it across the room at her sister.

It didn't hit Sierra, though. Instead, it hit the model city Sierra was building for a social studies project. Tiny, cardboard houses went scattering across the floor.

"Mom!" Sierra shrieked. "Mom!"

Patti flopped back on her bed and waited for their mother to come deal with the situation. She looked at her plump legs, the curve of her tummy, and she wished she could crawl out of her body and hide. She was so fat, she couldn't even throw a pillow the right way!

Why did she have to be so fat?

And why was Sierra so skinny?

WHERE IT ALL BEGINS: CALORIES

People are fat or skinny for a whole bunch of reasons. But the story starts with calories.

You've probably heard people talk about calories. Sometimes it may sound as though calories are bad things.

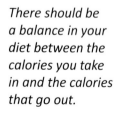

There should be a balance in your diet between the calories you take in and the calories that go out.

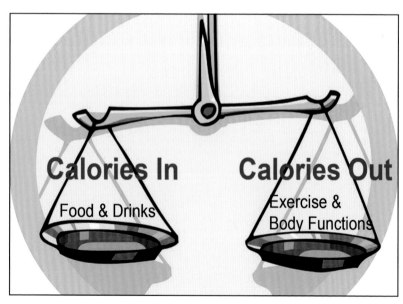

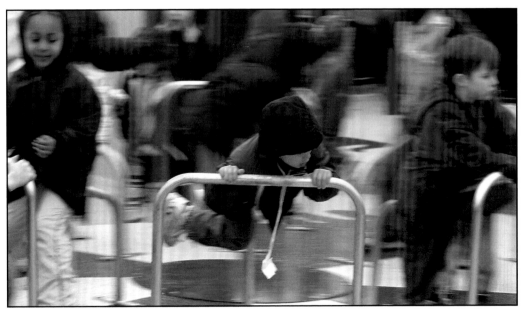

The calories you get from food and drinks give you the energy you need to play.

After all, commercials are always making low-calorie foods sound as though they're healthier, and people who are on a diet will often count calories. It's true that too many calories can make us fat—but we also need calories.

Calories are a way to measure what's in the food we eat. We use inches and feet (or centimeters and meters) to measure how long or tall something is; we use pints and quarts (or liters) to measure liquids like milk and soda. And we use calories to measure how much **energy** is in a certain food.

What is energy?
Energy is the ability to be active, the power it takes to move your body.

Each one of us needs a certain amount of calories every day to be healthy and have the energy we need for all the things we do in a day. Even sitting still takes a certain number of calories, but the more active we are, the more calories we need. People who are bigger, more active, or who are growing usually need more calories than smaller people, people who don't move around very much, and people who aren't growing.

When we eat more calories than we need, our bodies store the extra energy as fat. Long ago, our ancestors went through times when they had plenty of food, followed by times when food was scarcer.

If you eat more calories than your body needs, the extra energy will be stored as fat.

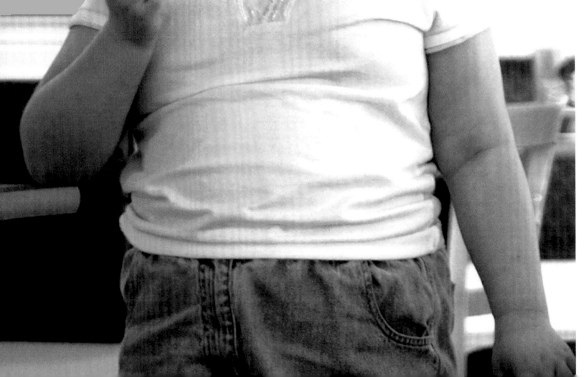

Their bodies' stores of fat helped them get through the times when they had less food. Today, though, many times our bodies just keep storing more and more fat that never needs to be used. When that happens, we end up being overweight or obese.

Everybody has different calorie needs.

Recommended Daily Calories		
Age	Boys	Girls
2	1000	1000
3	1000–1400	1000–1200
4–5	1200–1400	1200–1400
6	1400–1600	1200–1400
7	1400–1600	1200–1600
8	1400–1600	1400–1600
9	1600–1800	1400–1600
10	1600–1800	1400–1800
11	1800–2000	1600–1800
12	1800–2200	1600–2000
13	2000–2200	1600–2000
14	2000–2400	1800–2000
15	2200–2600	1800–2000
16–18	2400–2800	1800–2000
19–20	2600–2800	2000–2200

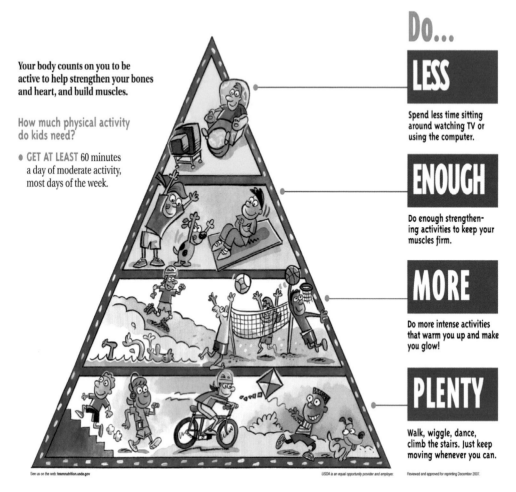

Your body counts on you to be active to help strengthen your bones and heart, and build muscles.

How much physical activity do kids need?

● GET AT LEAST 60 minutes a day of moderate activity, most days of the week.

Do...

LESS

Spend less time sitting around watching TV or using the computer.

ENOUGH

Do enough strengthening activities to keep your muscles firm.

MORE

Do more intense activities that warm you up and make you glow!

PLENTY

Walk, wiggle, dance, climb the stairs. Just keep moving whenever you can.

See us on the web: teamnutrition.usda.gov   USDA is an equal opportunity provider and employer.   Reviewed and approved for reprinting December 2007.

Getting more exercise is one way to burn more calories.

To get rid of these extra stores of fat, we need to do one of two things: take in fewer calories, forcing our bodies to use up the stored energy in our fat—or use up more calories by exercising more, which will also make our bodies use up the fat we've stored.

BUT IT'S NOT THAT SIMPLE: DIFFERENT KINDS OF BODIES

What's a gene? A gene is a tiny code inside the cells of our bodies. Together, all the genes in our cells are like a set of directions that tell our bodies what to look like (Will we have blue eyes or brown? Black hair or blonde? Brown skin or pink skin? Will we be short or tall?); what problems we might have (Will we have a certain disease? Will we have a hard time learning?), what our strengths will be (Will we be good at sports? Learn to play musical instruments easily? Draw well?); and whether we will be a boy or a girl. These "codes" are passed along from parents to their children.

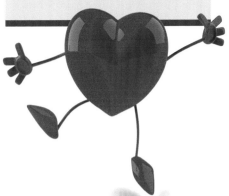

People's bodies are made differently. Even two sisters like Patti and Sierra may have different things inside their bodies that make their bodies deal with food differently.

Scientists have found that there's a special **gene** that some people have and some people don't. The people who have it can eat as much as they want. The calories they eat get turned into energy. People who don't have this gene—and that's most of us—will gain weight if they overeat. The extra calories they take in get turned into fat.

Scientists believe that other genes may also have a role in whether people are fat or thin. For instance, some people may simply feel hungry more often because of different **genetic** makeup.

Researchers don't believe that genes are the whole story, though, at least not in most cases. In other words, having a certain kind of gene or not having it will not automatically guarantee that you will be fat or skinny. Other things in our lives also play a role in whether we are overweight or obese.

There are inside-your-body reasons for gaining weight—but there are also outside-your-body reasons.

Your DNA helps decide your body type, but it is not the only factor.

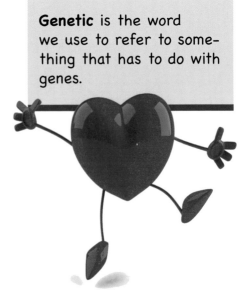

Genetic is the word we use to refer to something that has to do with genes.

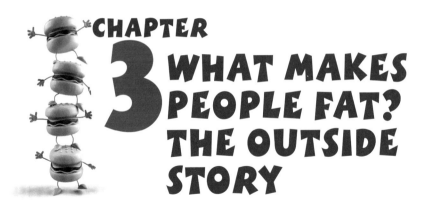

CHAPTER 3
WHAT MAKES PEOPLE FAT? THE OUTSIDE STORY

"I'm starving," Patti announced to her mother after her piano lesson.

"Me too," said Sierra.

"Me too," their mother said. "And I don't feel like going home to make dinner. Let's go through the drive-thru and get some fast food."

On Thursdays, their mom picked up the two girls after school and drove them to their lessons. Afterward, it would

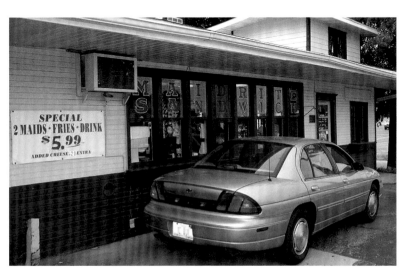

Drive through windows are a fast way to grab food when you are hungry, but do not have much time.

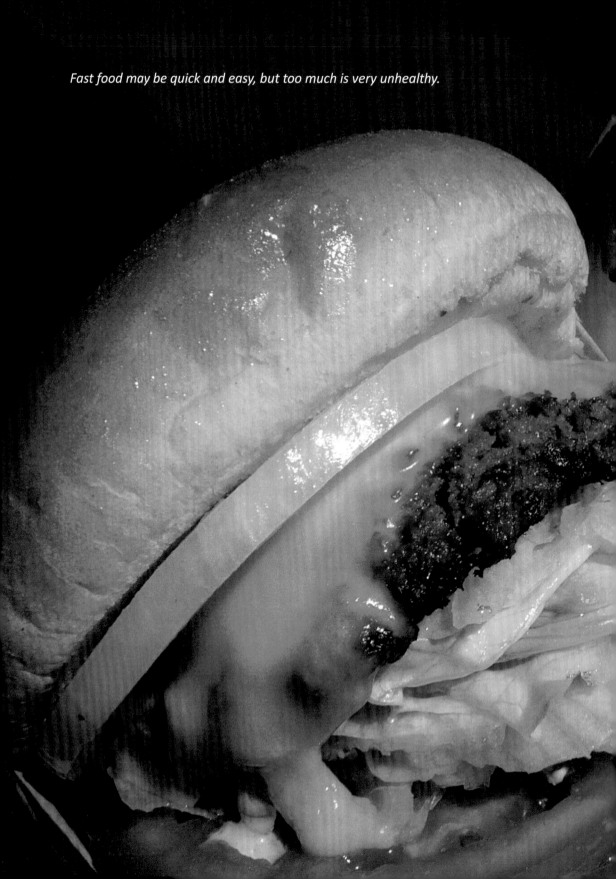

Fast food may be quick and easy, but too much is very unhealthy.

be time for supper, and all three of them were always hungry and grouchy. Most of the time, they stopped at one of their favorite fast-food restaurants on their way home.

Patti had been hoping that's what would happen tonight. She really truly couldn't wait to eat—and her favorite meal in the whole world was a cheeseburger, french fries, and a chocolate milkshake.

Many modern families are too busy to sit down to a family dinner at home every night. Fast food offers a quick and convenient option for families on the go.

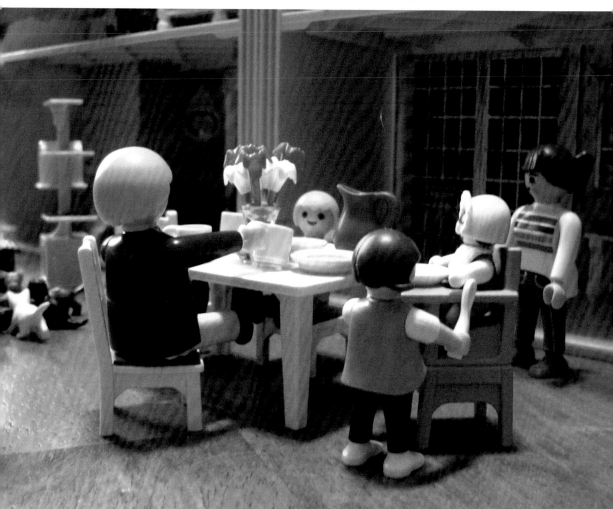

She bounced impatiently on the back seat while her mom placed their order at the drive-thru window. When her mother pulled the car forward to the next window, the sack full of hot food and the container of drinks were already waiting for them.

DID YOU KNOW?

A study of children who were six to eight years old found that 70 percent of them believed fast food was healthier than home-cooked food.

Her mom handed back burgers and drinks to the two girls. Patti and Sierra happily sucked on their straws. They played with the toys from their kids' meals and laughed. Sierra made hers talk in a silly voice, and Patti made hers answer.

Their mom laughed at the girls. "It's nice to hear you two getting along again."

She pulled in their driveway, and as they got out of the car, she said, "But tomorrow we really have to eat at home instead. And we have to have something healthy—that means vegetables!"

Patti made a face. Eating fast food was so much more fun than sitting around the table at home eating healthy food.

She followed Sierra into the living room and plopped down on the sofa to watch their favorite television show.

Food Survey of Children, Ages 2 to 9
Two-Day Survey (2002)

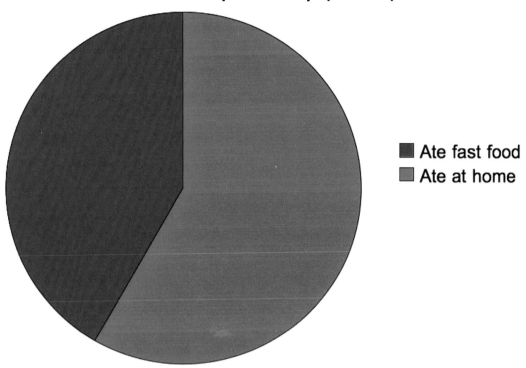

■ Ate fast food
■ Ate at home

Researchers have found that many children eat fast food a lot. This chart shows that almost half of children asked had eaten fast food two days in a row.

"Don't worry," Sierra whispered during the first commercial. "Mom always says that on piano lesson nights. But I bet we have pizza tomorrow."

Patti nodded.

"Mom," she called, "can we make popcorn?"

HOW OUR WORLD MAKES US FAT
THE FOOD WE EAT

Patti's family is no different from many others around the world. Like lots of families, they're busy, and they're in a hurry. Fast food has become an easy and convenient way to eat a meal.

A hundred years ago, families had different **traditions**. Most mothers stayed home and cooked the families' meals from scratch.

What are traditions? They're patterns of thinking or ways of doing things that are passed along from generation to generation.

Not only are children eating a lot of fast food, but they are getting less exercise.

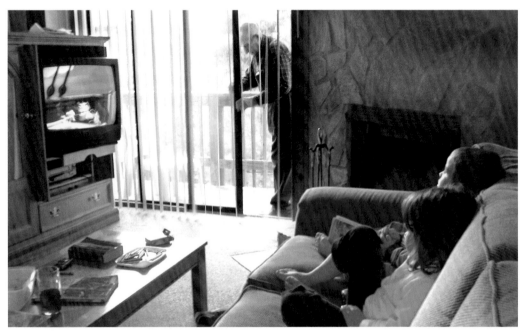

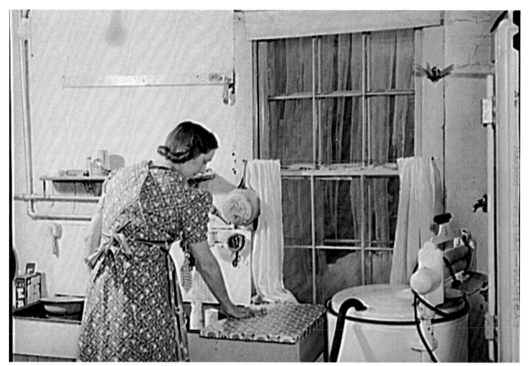

In the past, most mothers stayed home and were able to spend a lot of time making dinner every day.

Many families raised their own food. Food preparation took up a large part of every family's day. Children usually came home right after school, where they were expected to do their chores—help make supper, take care of the animals that provided food for the family, and do other food-related work.

DID YOU KNOW?

A recent study found that 89 percent of all children younger than eight years old visited McDonald's at least once a month.

Today, lots of mothers work outside the home, and most families are busy with many things: music lessons, sports practices, ballet lessons, and other after-school activities. It's hard to find time to prepare meals, and even when families do eat at home, they often rely on pre-packaged meals that are fast and easy to prepare.

Children today are lucky to have more opportunities than children in the past. Rather than just doing chores, kids today get to do things like play sports or learn piano.

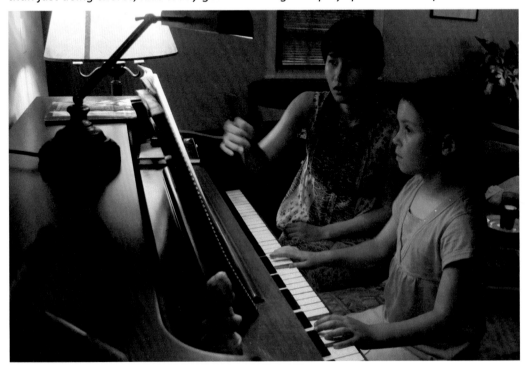

There are lots of reasons for the changes in our world today, and many of them are good things. For instance, it's a good thing that women today have more opportunities to do satisfying work than they did a hundred years ago. And participating in sports, music, and other activities can be good for kids. Having more time in our lives for the things we enjoy is a good thing too.

But the fast-food business has taken advantage of our changing lifestyles by selling us food that tastes good, is ready right away—and is full of things that have lots of calories, like sugar and fat. The packaged foods we often eat at home are also often full of sugar and fat. But we've gotten used to the taste of fast foods and packaged foods. Many children prefer them.

Today's serving sizes are much bigger than your grandmother's were. When we pull up at a drive-thru window, we've come to expect big cups of soda and huge sandwiches. Even our kids' meals are bigger than they used to be. In fact, most adult-size meals were once the size of what kids' meals are today.

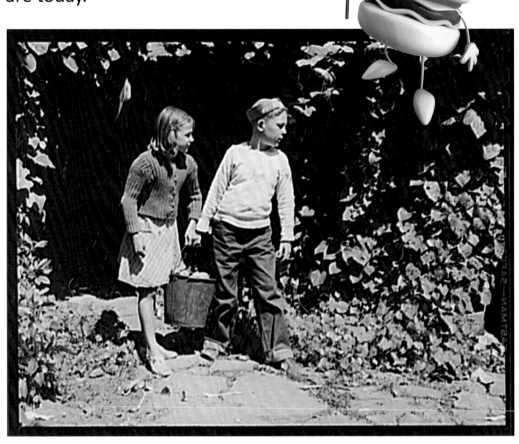

In the past, the chores that children had to help with every day helped burn a lot of calories. Today, children spend more time sitting around playing video games or watching T.V.

All these changes in the world where we live make it harder than it once was to eat a healthy diet. We end up eating more calories than our bodies need. Our eating habits help make more and more of us over-weight.

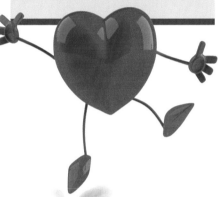

What does sedentary mean? It means that you spend most of your time sitting down, not moving around or exercising.

PLUS WE DON'T EXERCISE

Those chores your grandparents did after school may not have been a lot of fun—but they were hard work that burned a lot of calories. When kids a hundred years ago weren't working, they were playing games like hopscotch and jump rope, hide-and-seek and keep-away—games that also burned a lot of calories.

What do most kids do today when they're at home? Like Patti, they watch television. (And a lot of the time, they eat snacks while they do.) Or they play computer games. Or they listen to music on their iPods or MP3 players. Our world is full of electronic devices your grandparents never dreamed of. These inventions are truly wonderful in many ways—but they also encourage us all, children and grownups alike, to have **sedentary** lifestyles.

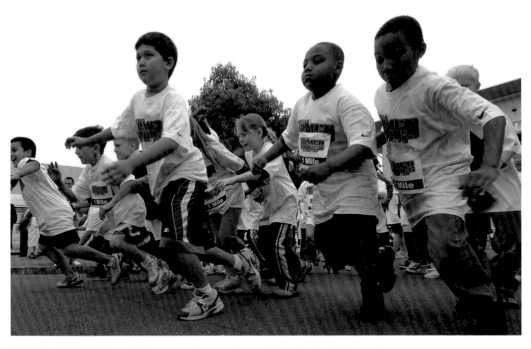

Kids (and adults) need to stay active to burn the calories they eat.

When we spend so much time sitting down (whether we're watching television or playing a computer game), we don't burn as many calories. So not only are we taking in more calories in the food we eat, we're also not using as many calories.

And all those things help to make more and more children and adults either overweight or obese.

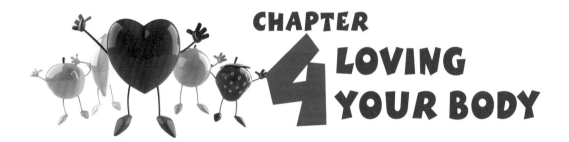

CHAPTER 4
LOVING YOUR BODY

"Come on, Miss Piggy," called Jeremy, Patti and Sierra's babysitter. "Time for bed. Turn off the TV and get into your PJs."

"Don't call me that!" Patti glared up at Jeremy.

Jeremy looked surprised. "But I've always called you that, Patti. Ever since you were little."

Friends love joking around and laughing together, but sometimes the wrong jokes can be hurtful.

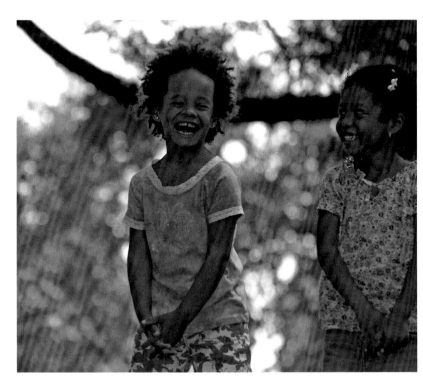

"Well, I don't like it. It's a mean name."

"I'm sorry, Patti. But you have those big eyes and long eye-lashes, just like Miss Piggy does."

"And I'm fat."

Jeremy looked uncomfortable. "I'm sorry," he said again. "I was just teasing you, I guess. I didn't want to be mean to you."

Patti signed. She liked Jeremy, and she didn't want to make him feel sad. "I'm tired of being teased," she said softly.

Later that night, when she heard her mom come home, Patti got up from her bed quietly, careful not to disturb Sierra. She waited until she heard Jeremy leave, and then she tiptoed down the stairs. "Mom?"

Her mother looked up at her. "What is it, Patti? Why aren't you in bed?"

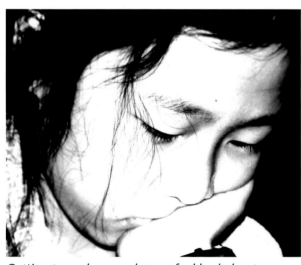

Getting teased can make you feel bad about yourself.

Patti crawled onto the sofa next to her mother and leaned against her. "I couldn't sleep. I was thinking."

Her mother put her arm around Patti.

"What were you thinking about?"

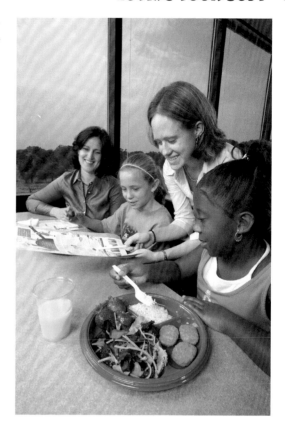

A nutritionist or dietician can help teach you what to eat and how to keep your body its healthiest.

"I was thinking that I'm tired of being fat. I'm tired of being teased." She tipped her head up to looking into her mom's face. "Is there anything I can do about it?"

Her mom looked back at her for a long moment. Then she nodded. "I'll make an appointment with Dr. Narby. We'll ask her advice about what you can do to lose weight. And I'll help you. It's not your fault, you know, Patti."

"It must be my fault," Patti insisted. "Sierra's not fat. But I am. I'm lazy and I eat too much."

Her mom shook her head. "No, it's not your fault, Patti. It's partly my fault. And it's partly just the way you're made. Sierra is always going to have a tall, thin body, and you're always going to be shorter and more stocky. But you're each beautiful in your own way, you really, really are, Patti.

The only thing that matters is being healthy. I want you to be the best you that you can possibly be—and I want you to know how wonderful you are, Patti, how absolutely gorgeous and pretty and amazing you truly are!"

IT'S A QUESTION OF HEALTH

Between the inside-the-body story and the outside-the-body story, kids like Patti who are overweight really can't blame themselves. Being overweight or obese is a big problem, and many people share this problem around the world. But it's a health problem, not a problem that's caused by people being bad or lazy or stupid.

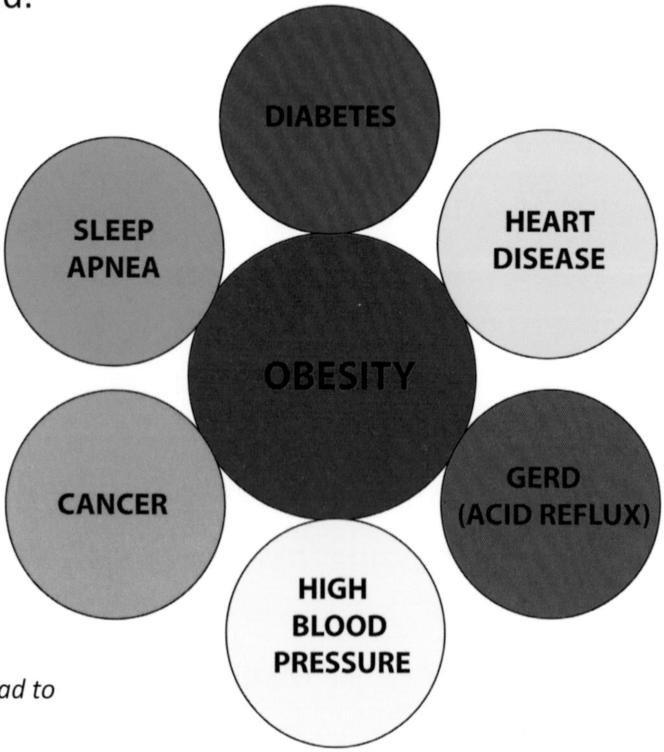

DIABETES

SLEEP APNEA

HEART DISEASE

OBESITY

CANCER

GERD (ACID REFLUX)

HIGH BLOOD PRESSURE

Obesity and overweight are health problems that can lead to other health problems.

Adults around the world are searching for the answers to this problem. Scientists, doctors, teachers, government leaders, and parents are all working to figure out ways to change both the inside story and the outside story. They are looking for ways to make the world where we live a place where it's easier to eat a healthy diet and exercise more.

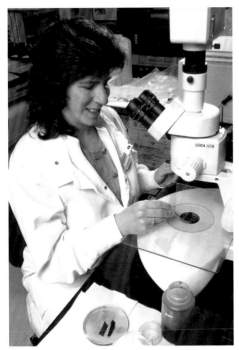

Many scientists are working to learn more about the causes of obesity.

YOUR AMAZING BODY

In the meantime, hating your own body will not help you lose weight. It will just make you sad and discouraged and angry— and all those feelings may actually make you eat more, and gain still more weight. Children and adults who are overweight or obese need to love their bodies.

Lots of people today think that there's only one kind of pretty—the very skinny, tall kind of pretty you see on magazine covers. But that's not true. The human body comes in a lot of shapes and sizes. Some people are naturally tall and thin. Others are shorter and thicker.

Whether we're fat or thin is just one very small piece of who we are. But all healthy bodies do all sorts of amazing things. They can run and jump, see and smell, laugh and talk. They express our feelings. They allow us to play. They let us build things and paint things and write stories.

The most important thing is to love who you are. If you do, you'll want to take as good care of your body as you can. That means keeping it as healthy as you can.

MAKING YOUR OWN CHOICES

Just because you're a kid doesn't mean you can't make important choices about your life. You can begin to choose what kinds of food you eat. In fact, you've probably been doing that since you were very young! You can also help the grownups in your life think more about eating healthier foods and exercising more.

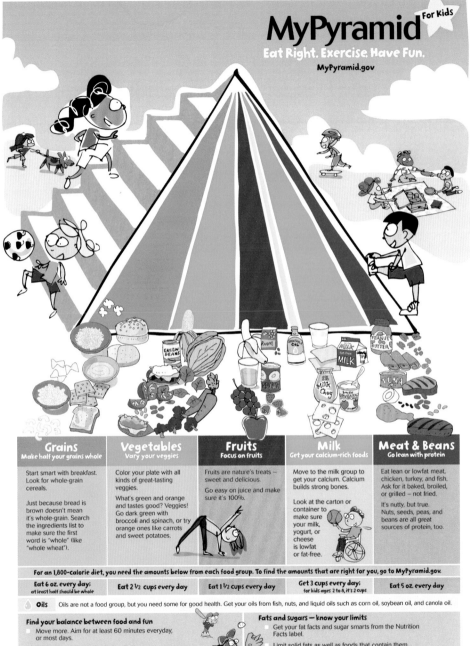

MyPyramid For Kids
Eat Right. Exercise. Have Fun.
MyPyramid.gov

Grains	**Vegetables**	**Fruits**	**Milk**	**Meat & Beans**
Make half your grains whole	Vary your veggies	Focus on fruits	Get your calcium-rich foods	Go lean with protein
Start smart with breakfast. Look for whole-grain cereals. Just because bread is brown doesn't mean it's whole-grain. Search the ingredients list to make sure the first word is "whole" (like "whole wheat").	Color your plate with all kinds of great-tasting veggies. What's green and orange and tastes good? Veggies! Go dark green with broccoli and spinach, or try orange ones like carrots and sweet potatoes.	Fruits are nature's treats — sweet and delicious. Go easy on juice and make sure it's 100%.	Move to the milk group to get your calcium. Calcium builds strong bones. Look at the carton or container to make sure your milk, yogurt, or cheese is lowfat or fat-free.	Eat lean or lowfat meat, chicken, turkey, and fish. Ask for it baked, broiled, or grilled — not fried. It's nutty, but true. Nuts, seeds, peas, and beans are all great sources of protein, too.

For an 1,800-calorie diet, you need the amounts below from each food group. To find the amounts that are right for you, go to MyPyramid.gov.

Eat 6 oz. every day; at least half should be whole	Eat 2 ½ cups every day	Eat 1 ½ cups every day	Get 3 cups every day; for kids ages 2 to 8, it's 2 cups	Eat 5 oz. every day

Oils Oils are not a food group, but you need some for good health. Get your oils from fish, nuts, and liquid oils such as corn oil, soybean oil, and canola oil.

Find your balance between food and fun
- Move more. Aim for at least 60 minutes everyday, or most days.
- Walk, dance, bike, rollerblade – it all counts. How great is that!

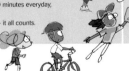

Fats and sugars — know your limits
- Get your fat facts and sugar smarts from the Nutrition Facts label.
- Limit solid fats as well as foods that contain them.
- Choose food and beverages low in added sugars and other caloric sweeteners.

MyPyramid.gov
STEPS TO A HEALTHIER YOU

U.S. Department of Agriculture
Food and Nutrition Service
September 2005
FNS-387

USDA is an equal opportunity provider and employer

You have power! You can choose to take care of your body by giving it healthy food and plenty of exercise. You can influence your family to exercise more and eat better.

And as you get older, you're going to have more and more control over you life. Even though you are a kid, you can make choices today that will shape who you become as an adult. If you look at your parents, you'll probably notice they don't do things the same way your grandparents do. They've made choices about their lives that are all their own. You'll have the chance to do the same.

The food you choose to eat is an important way to choose who you want to be. Each time you put something in your mouth, take time to think about it. Think about what you really want to eat.

Love yourself enough to shape healthy habits that will last a lifetime.

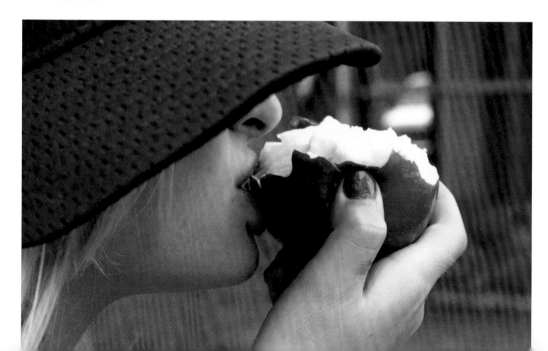

READ MORE ABOUT IT

Abramovitz, Melissa. *Diseases & Disorders: Obesity.* Farmington Hills, Mich.: Lucent, 2004.

Chilman-Blair, Kim. *What's Up with Pam?* New York: Rosen, 2010.

Gay, Kathlyn. *Am I Fat?* Berkeley Heights, N.J.: Enslow, 2006.

Jimerson, M. N. *Childhood Obesity.* Farmington Hills, Mich.: Lucent, 2008.

Johnson, Susan and Laurel Mellin. *Just for Kids! Obesity Prevention.* San Anselmo, Calif.: Balboa, 2002.

Olson, Judith K. *I Can Hardly Wait.* Parker, Colo.: Outskirts, 2006.

Prim-Ed. *Lifestyle Choices.* Boston: Prim-Ed, 2005.

Watson, Stephanie. *The Genetics of Obesity.* New York: Rosen, 2008.

FIND OUT MORE ON THE INTERNET

Comfort Eating
www.blubberbuster.com/board/
emotional_eating.htm

Emotional Eating
kidshealth.org/teen/food_fitness/
dieting/emotional_eating.html

Empowered Kids
www.treatingeatingdisorders.com/
empoweredkidz/

Family Food Experts
betterfoodchoices.info

The Food Guide Pyramid
kidshealth.org/kid/stay_healthy/food/
pyramid.html

Healthy Food Choices: Nutrition
Explorations
www.nutritionexplorations.org/parents/
health-food.asp

MyPyramid for Kids
www.mypyramid.gov/Kids/

The websites listed on this page were active at the time of publication. The publisher is not responsible for websites that have changed their address or discontinued operation since the date of publication. The publisher will review and update the websites upon each reprint.

INDEX

PICTURE CREDITS

ABOUT THE AUTHOR

Jamie Hunt is a certified teacher who has taught health to children from eleven to thirteen years old. She has worked with many publishers on a number of health-related books for young people. She lives in New York State.